INFORMATION

MW00475870

NAME	
Registration Details	
Work Address:	

Phone No.		**Email**	
Fax No.		**Emergency No.**	
Website			
Log Book Number			

Continued From Log Book:		**Continued To Log Book:**	
Date Log Started:		**Date Log Ended:**	

NOTES

_____
_____
_____
_____
_____
_____
_____
_____
_____
_____
_____
_____
_____

INDEX

PAGE NUMBER	CLIENT
1	
2	
3	
4	
5	
6	
7	
8	
9	
10	
11	
12	
13	
14	
15	
16	
17	
18	
19	
20	
21	
22	
23	
24	
25	

INDEX

PAGE NUMBER	CLIENT
26	
27	
28	
29	
30	
31	
32	
33	
34	
35	
36	
37	
38	
39	
40	
41	
42	
43	
44	
45	
46	
47	
48	
49	
50	

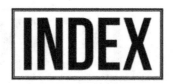

INDEX

PAGE NUMBER	CLIENT
51	
52	
53	
54	
55	
56	
57	
58	
59	
60	
61	
62	
63	
64	
65	
66	
67	
68	
69	
70	
71	
72	
73	
74	
75	

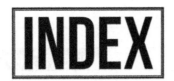

INDEX

PAGE NUMBER	CLIENT
76	
77	
78	
79	
80	
81	
82	
83	
84	
85	
86	
87	
88	
89	
90	
91	
92	
93	
94	
95	
96	
97	
98	
99	
100	

CLIENT LOG

CLIENT NAME

DATE

NEXT APPOINTMENT

ACTIONS

CLIENT LOG

CLIENT NAME

DATE | **NEXT APPOINTMENT**

ACTIONS

CLIENT LOG

CLIENT NAME

DATE   **NEXT APPOINTMENT**

ACTIONS

CLIENT NAME

DATE   NEXT APPOINTMENT

ACTIONS

CLIENT LOG

CLIENT NAME

DATE   **NEXT APPOINTMENT**

ACTIONS

CLIENT NAME

DATE   **NEXT APPOINTMENT**

ACTIONS

CLIENT LOG

CLIENT NAME

DATE   NEXT APPOINTMENT

ACTIONS

CLIENT NAME

DATE

NEXT APPOINTMENT

ACTIONS

CLIENT LOG

CLIENT NAME

DATE   **NEXT APPOINTMENT**

ACTIONS

CLIENT NAME

DATE   NEXT APPOINTMENT

ACTIONS

CLIENT LOG

CLIENT NAME

DATE　　　　　　　　　　　　　　　　**NEXT APPOINTMENT**

ACTIONS

CLIENT NAME

DATE   NEXT APPOINTMENT

ACTIONS

CLIENT LOG

CLIENT NAME

DATE

NEXT APPOINTMENT

ACTIONS

CLIENT NAME

DATE   **NEXT APPOINTMENT**

ACTIONS

CLIENT LOG

CLIENT NAME

DATE   **NEXT APPOINTMENT**

ACTIONS

CLIENT NAME

DATE   NEXT APPOINTMENT

ACTIONS

CLIENT LOG

CLIENT NAME

DATE   NEXT APPOINTMENT

ACTIONS

CLIENT LOG

CLIENT NAME

DATE   **NEXT APPOINTMENT**

ACTIONS

CLIENT LOG

CLIENT NAME

DATE

NEXT APPOINTMENT

ACTIONS

CLIENT NAME

DATE   NEXT APPOINTMENT

ACTIONS

CLIENT LOG

CLIENT NAME

DATE

NEXT APPOINTMENT

ACTIONS

CLIENT LOG

CLIENT NAME

DATE

NEXT APPOINTMENT

ACTIONS

CLIENT LOG

CLIENT NAME

DATE   **NEXT APPOINTMENT**

ACTIONS

CLIENT NAME

DATE

NEXT APPOINTMENT

ACTIONS

CLIENT LOG

CLIENT NAME

DATE   **NEXT APPOINTMENT**

ACTIONS

CLIENT NAME

DATE   NEXT APPOINTMENT

ACTIONS

CLIENT LOG

CLIENT NAME

DATE   NEXT APPOINTMENT

ACTIONS

CLIENT NAME

DATE   **NEXT APPOINTMENT**

ACTIONS

CLIENT LOG

CLIENT NAME

DATE

NEXT APPOINTMENT

ACTIONS

CLIENT LOG

CLIENT NAME

DATE

NEXT APPOINTMENT

ACTIONS

CLIENT LOG

CLIENT NAME

DATE   **NEXT APPOINTMENT**

ACTIONS

CLIENT NAME

DATE   NEXT APPOINTMENT

ACTIONS

CLIENT LOG

CLIENT NAME

DATE

NEXT APPOINTMENT

ACTIONS

CLIENT NAME

DATE   NEXT APPOINTMENT

ACTIONS

CLIENT LOG

CLIENT NAME

DATE

NEXT APPOINTMENT

ACTIONS

CLIENT LOG

CLIENT NAME

DATE   NEXT APPOINTMENT

ACTIONS

CLIENT LOG

CLIENT NAME

DATE   **NEXT APPOINTMENT**

ACTIONS

CLIENT NAME

DATE

NEXT APPOINTMENT

ACTIONS

CLIENT LOG

CLIENT NAME

DATE   NEXT APPOINTMENT

ACTIONS

CLIENT NAME

DATE

NEXT APPOINTMENT

ACTIONS

CLIENT LOG

CLIENT NAME

DATE   NEXT APPOINTMENT

ACTIONS

CLIENT NAME

DATE　　　　　　　　　　　　　　　　　　　**NEXT APPOINTMENT**

ACTIONS

42

CLIENT LOG

CLIENT NAME

DATE

NEXT APPOINTMENT

ACTIONS

CLIENT LOG

CLIENT NAME

DATE   **NEXT APPOINTMENT**

ACTIONS

CLIENT LOG

CLIENT NAME

DATE   **NEXT APPOINTMENT**

ACTIONS

CLIENT NAME

DATE

NEXT APPOINTMENT

ACTIONS

CLIENT LOG

CLIENT NAME

DATE

NEXT APPOINTMENT

ACTIONS

CLIENT NAME

DATE   **NEXT APPOINTMENT**

ACTIONS

CLIENT LOG

CLIENT NAME

DATE   **NEXT APPOINTMENT**

ACTIONS

CLIENT NAME

DATE   NEXT APPOINTMENT

ACTIONS

CLIENT LOG

CLIENT NAME

DATE   NEXT APPOINTMENT

ACTIONS

CLIENT LOG

CLIENT NAME

DATE **NEXT APPOINTMENT**

ACTIONS

CLIENT LOG

CLIENT NAME

DATE   NEXT APPOINTMENT

ACTIONS

CLIENT NAME

DATE   NEXT APPOINTMENT

ACTIONS

CLIENT LOG

CLIENT NAME

DATE

NEXT APPOINTMENT

ACTIONS

CLIENT NAME

DATE   NEXT APPOINTMENT

ACTIONS

CLIENT LOG

CLIENT NAME

DATE   **NEXT APPOINTMENT**

ACTIONS

CLIENT LOG

CLIENT NAME

DATE

NEXT APPOINTMENT

ACTIONS

CLIENT LOG

CLIENT NAME

DATE

NEXT APPOINTMENT

ACTIONS

CLIENT NAME

DATE　　　　　　　　　　　　　　　**NEXT APPOINTMENT**

ACTIONS

CLIENT LOG

CLIENT NAME

DATE   **NEXT APPOINTMENT**

ACTIONS

CLIENT NAME

DATE   NEXT APPOINTMENT

ACTIONS

CLIENT LOG

CLIENT NAME

DATE

NEXT APPOINTMENT

ACTIONS

CLIENT NAME

DATE | **NEXT APPOINTMENT**

ACTIONS

CLIENT LOG

CLIENT NAME

DATE

NEXT APPOINTMENT

ACTIONS

CLIENT LOG

CLIENT NAME

DATE   NEXT APPOINTMENT

ACTIONS

CLIENT LOG

CLIENT NAME

DATE

NEXT APPOINTMENT

ACTIONS

CLIENT NAME

DATE   NEXT APPOINTMENT

ACTIONS

CLIENT LOG

CLIENT NAME

DATE

NEXT APPOINTMENT

ACTIONS

CLIENT LOG

CLIENT NAME

DATE

NEXT APPOINTMENT

ACTIONS

CLIENT LOG

CLIENT NAME

DATE　　　　　　　　　　　　　　　**NEXT APPOINTMENT**

ACTIONS

CLIENT LOG

CLIENT NAME

DATE   **NEXT APPOINTMENT**

ACTIONS

CLIENT LOG

CLIENT NAME

DATE

NEXT APPOINTMENT

ACTIONS

CLIENT LOG

CLIENT NAME

DATE   NEXT APPOINTMENT

ACTIONS

CLIENT LOG

CLIENT NAME

DATE

NEXT APPOINTMENT

ACTIONS

CLIENT NAME

DATE | **NEXT APPOINTMENT**

ACTIONS

CLIENT LOG

CLIENT NAME

DATE   **NEXT APPOINTMENT**

ACTIONS

CLIENT LOG

CLIENT NAME

DATE   **NEXT APPOINTMENT**

ACTIONS

CLIENT LOG

CLIENT NAME

DATE   NEXT APPOINTMENT

ACTIONS

CLIENT LOG

CLIENT NAME

DATE   **NEXT APPOINTMENT**

ACTIONS

CLIENT LOG

CLIENT NAME

DATE   **NEXT APPOINTMENT**

ACTIONS

CLIENT NAME

DATE   **NEXT APPOINTMENT**

ACTIONS

CLIENT LOG

CLIENT NAME

DATE   **NEXT APPOINTMENT**

ACTIONS

CLIENT LOG

CLIENT NAME

DATE   NEXT APPOINTMENT

ACTIONS

CLIENT LOG

CLIENT NAME

DATE

NEXT APPOINTMENT

ACTIONS

CLIENT NAME

DATE

NEXT APPOINTMENT

ACTIONS

CLIENT LOG

CLIENT NAME

DATE   NEXT APPOINTMENT

ACTIONS

CLIENT NAME

DATE NEXT APPOINTMENT

ACTIONS

CLIENT LOG

CLIENT NAME

DATE   **NEXT APPOINTMENT**

ACTIONS

CLIENT NAME

DATE   NEXT APPOINTMENT

ACTIONS

CLIENT LOG

CLIENT NAME

DATE

NEXT APPOINTMENT

ACTIONS

CLIENT NAME

DATE

NEXT APPOINTMENT

ACTIONS

CLIENT LOG

CLIENT NAME

DATE

NEXT APPOINTMENT

ACTIONS

CLIENT LOG

CLIENT NAME

DATE

NEXT APPOINTMENT

ACTIONS

CLIENT LOG

CLIENT NAME

DATE

NEXT APPOINTMENT

ACTIONS

CLIENT NAME

DATE

NEXT APPOINTMENT

ACTIONS

CLIENT LOG

CLIENT NAME

DATE

NEXT APPOINTMENT

ACTIONS

CLIENT LOG

CLIENT NAME

DATE   NEXT APPOINTMENT

ACTIONS

CLIENT LOG

CLIENT NAME

DATE   NEXT APPOINTMENT

ACTIONS

CLIENT NAME

DATE　　　　　　　　　　　　　　**NEXT APPOINTMENT**

ACTIONS